Estheticians are a Girl's Best Friend

DIANE BUCCOLA

DEDICATION

To professional Estheticians everywhere who work tirelessly to achieve higher esthetic education and perfect their skills in order to better care for their clients.

CONTENTS

(Es-the-tish-uhn) *n.*

A person skilled in the art of skin care treatments; facials, waxing; well-versed in the subject of skin care and maintenance.

A smart individual who has contracted a case of skin health sense and is determined to spread the condition.

Synonyms: *Aesthetician, skin care goddess, facial diva, sunscreen queen, friend, secret-keeper, holder of the key to the Fountain of Youth.*

Common tools: *Fan brush, steamer, extractor, tweezers, wax sticks, magic wrinkle eraser.*

1. INTRODUCTION

2016 marks my 17th year as a licensed esthetician. During this time, not only have I seen the field of esthetics evolve dramatically, but I have learned a lot about women; specifically, the burdens they bear related to how they view themselves. While women are certainly concerned about good health and the art of aging gracefully, they do not always know where to go for solid information and accurate advice about skin care.

It has been my experience that women are quick to view their perceived "flaws" and will go to great and sometimes dangerous lengths to correct them. In fact, sometimes they will go from washing their face with nothing but bar soap, directly to surgery -- without even considering the plethora of less severe (and much safer) options that are available today. As estheticians, we are studied in the science of skin and aging, so we know that rarely are these actual "flaws." Rather, they are perceptions based upon how women measure themselves against the unrealistic standards suggested by media.

Women in particular are bombarded on a daily basis with TV and magazine ads promoting the latest and greatest in "anti-aging" and "anti-wrinkle" products. These commercials feature well-paid celebrities and beautiful models that have been perfected by a team of beauty professionals before their images are captured by masters of lighting and experts in photography. In some cases, the women in these ads have even been Photo-shopped or airbrushed to the point of perfection. So if you step back for a moment, you will realize the brainwashing and manipulation being used to motivate women to buy these products.

The Detox Challenge

Like many other women, I too was living under the spell of media's influence until one day a friend presented me with a challenge: For one week, whenever I was watching TV, I was to note all influences suggesting that perhaps I wasn't good enough as-is. It was an eye-opening experience for me! I saw so many commercials warning of physical impairments and medical conditions that we may have currently or could have in the future. There are ads for drugs we should take, and various cures we didn't know we needed for conditions we didn't know we had. There are body shaming ads, suggesting we need to lose weight, exercise more, or fix something. It is repeatedly suggested that we hide, remove, tighten and lift parts of our bodies. And those are just the TV commercials. (I won't even go into what we see on reality TV!)

Get factual information about your skin.

Ultimately what I learned from that week-long experiment is that we are mindlessly absorbing a lot of negative influences on a daily basis. It impacts our lives in ways we don't realize; especially for women, it sabotages our self-esteem. What appears simply to be an advertisement, is actually a suggestion. And that suggestion becomes a thought. And then, in our vulnerable mindset, that thought becomes a belief. And the next thing we know, we are looking to needles and scalpels to solve the "problem." My personal solution was to ignore these influences by simply hitting the mute button on my TV remote. This minimal effort has dramatically increased my self-awareness while decreasing my stress level. I highly recommend it.

Great skin can be simple and affordable. And that's why I have written this book, to provide general information to guide you through the world of high-tech and ever-evolving skin care. There are many skin care options available from multiple providers, in a variety of price ranges and intensity levels. There is literally a buffet of options to choose from which includes everything from products for home use, all the way to surgical services.

No matter what any manufacturer or the media tries to tell you, there is no anti-aging miracle product that will work for every woman. And *more expensive* does not mean *better*. We all have personal variables which determine how well our skin will age such as genetics, environmental exposure, lifestyle choices, hormones and health issues. And even within those parameters, much depends upon how the skin is maintained. Things will definitely shift throughout our lives, so each woman's optimal skin care protocol is specific to her and her alone.

My "A-ha" Moment

Throughout my many years as a professional esthetician, I have been exposed to women of all ages. And without fail, any time I am in a social situation and word gets out that I am an esthetician, I am inundated with skin care questions. I certainly don't mind discussing this because it is my favorite topic, but because I am a professional, I also know that there is only so much advice I can give outside of my treatment room. It would be irresponsible of me to recommend specific products without completing a proper intake process which includes a comprehensive skin evaluation.

I realized that this book needed to be written when I was asked to speak on the topic of skin care at a women's luncheon event. I had a short window of time allotted for my presentation, so I chose the topics that I have been asked about most often over the years, which at the time was sun damage and anti-aging. As I looked over the audience from my elevated perch, I could see that the 150 women in attendance were paying very close attention to my words; and to my surprise, the food servers had stopped working and were standing at the back of the room listening intently.

The ladies in the audience asked me so many questions that I ran out of time and got the signal from the host to wrap it up. I apologized for having to cut off the Q & A, and I offered to make myself available at the close of the event to answer more questions.

After the event ended, I continued the discussion for as long as I could, and was thanked profusely by these lovely women. The big lesson for me that day was that are so many women (and men) who really want to learn about good skin care and are willing to put in the effort to achieve their skin care goals, but unfortunately they're not sure how to accomplish this. They do try though, by purchasing products that they hear about from various sources. But unless they have personal access to a qualified esthetician, it is not likely that they are getting accurate information related to their specific needs.

As I exited the luncheon that day, I had an "a-ha" moment. I realized that although I couldn't personally absorb all of these women into my esthetics practice, I could at least help guide them through the maze of skin care options and provide them with information that they would not otherwise have access to; the goal being that they would find *their own perfect path* to great skin. So I left that day determined to get this information into the hands of as many women as possible. And this book was borne out of that commitment.

Bridging the Gap

I understand that not everyone has the time or budget to enjoy a monthly facial service. But today's estheticians do much more than simply give facials. They are trained in skin analysis, the science of skin and skin care, and they have a vast knowledge of products and ingredients. After a comprehensive consultation, an esthetician can guide you to home care products and protocols to get you started, and they can monitor results and make adjustments to meet your needs as things change throughout your life.

I think women need to support other women, and my favorite part of working as an esthetician has always been helping women look good and feel better about themselves. And that is my goal here. We all deserve to feel beautiful at any age, and I have written this book in an attempt to bridge the gap between estheticians and consumers.

I have chosen to focus primarily on women in this book because they tend to be the ones who are targeted by, and fall victim to, Over-The-Counter and Multi-Level-Marketing companies' false claims and broken promises. However, I have also addressed men's skin care in this book. It is becoming more and more important that women understand the dangerous impact that sun exposure is having on the men in their lives. For example, do you know that from age 50 on, significantly more men develop melanoma than women?[1] *(Please see Chapter 8 for more Skin Cancer Facts.)*

It takes a lot of time, training and dedication to become a qualified and really good esthetician; therefore, it would be irresponsible of me to put too much technical information in this book that could fall into the hands of unqualified interested parties (and there are SO many these days!). So once again, I urge you to find a qualified esthetician in your area so you can discover your personal path to optimum skin

---

[1] *www.SkinCancer.org*

health and reclaim -- and maintain -- your youthful appearance.

"I am going to make everything around me more beautiful.

That will be my life."

~ Elise de Wolfe

*I'm looking for a moisturizer
which will hide the fact
that I've been tired since 2010.*

2. HOW YOUNG ARE YOU?

What is the Skin?

The skin is the largest organ of the body. It covers the internal organs and protects them from injury, serves as a barrier between germs and internal organs, and prevents the loss of too much water and other fluids. The skin regulates body temperature and helps the body get rid of excess water and salts. Certain cells in the skin communicate with the brain and allow temperature, touch and pain sensations.

The Aging Process

The skin is influenced by both internal and external factors: From health, nutrition and genetics, to daily life habits and exercise, sun exposure and sleep. A person's apparent age depends upon genetics and how the skin is cared for on a regular basis.

The natural aging process -- the inevitable changes that are chronological -- is called *intrinsic* aging. In all people as we age, the rate at which the skin sheds old cells begins to slow, and the collagen and elastin network begin to degrade as expected with intrinsic aging.

Extrinsic aging, on the other hand, is environmental aging; the aging changes that are induced by UV radiation. The skin becomes rougher, elasticity is lost and wrinkling is increased. These visible signs of sun-related damage and hyperpigmentation are evident as *extrinsic* aging.

Sure...

you can sleep in your makeup,
smoke cigarettes,
not wear spf,
never get a facial,
and look 10 years younger.

Let me just grab my magic wand.

Your skin will be around a lot longer than that expensive handbag.

Invest in yourself.

3. PRODUCTS

The Good News
Skin care products have evolved over the years from bar soap and cold cream to professional products that can literally turn back the hands of time. The discovery and development of new active ingredients in skin care products has been amazing to watch during my career as an esthetician, and that is what has kept me in the business for so many years. It is to the esthetician's and consumer's benefit that manufacturers work very hard and spend lots of money to research and develop better and more results-oriented products in order to compete with each other.

The "Bad" News
It seems that everyone these days wants to be in the spa business. When I started my esthetics career, estheticians were found mostly in day spas, like mine. Throughout the years, however, I have seen many hair salons become "spas," along with every kind of doctor opening a "medi-spa" (aka, medical spa). Unfortunately, the average consumer assumes that if a doctor is attached to it, it must be good or at least better. (More aggressive? *Probably*. Better? *Not necessarily.*)

Consumers are bombarded with skin care advice via television commercials and magazines. More often than not, the products recommended are over-the-counter products that are super-expensive and are sold by salespeople who are not qualified to analyze a client's skin properly or accurately recommend products. And even if these salespeople were somehow qualified, over-the-counter products are never going to be as effective as professional-grade products recommended by a trained, licensed and qualified esthetician who has carefully evaluated the current condition of a client's skin. And sadly, consumers unknowingly pour their hard-earned money into products that really are not going to produce the results they are hoping for.

OTC and MLM v. Pro

I always ask new clients to give me their opinion of their skin. And I very often find that a client who says her skin is dry is almost always using Over-The-Counter (OTC)[2] or Multi-Level-Marketing (MLM)[3] products that are not suitable for her. Clients often mistakenly believe that there is something wrong with their skin rather than considering the more likely cause that the products they are currently using are incorrect.

For example, if you are using a cleanser that lathers and therefore cuts through the skin's natural oil, and a moisturizer that does not have appropriate ingredients to ensure re-hydration, of course your skin will feel dry. I once did a study on a well-known bar soap (that was often handed out by many dermatologists to their patients). My research showed that the ingredient list included 7 different detergents, which means 7 times more likely to dry out your skin!

---

[2] *Over-The-Counter skin care products typically sold at department stores, drug stores, grocery stores, etc.*

[3] *Multi-Level-Marketing (pyramid) products sold by way of home parties, door-to-door, catalogs, etc., by non- professionals.*

Another example is a client who feels oily or is breaking out. For a woman struggling with these issues, very often she is using a moisturizer that is too rich and emollient for her current skin condition and may not be exfoliating properly. In other words, perhaps these products and protocols made sense at one time in her life, but things change.

And although men's skin tends to be oilier than women's (which is not necessarily a bad thing as far as aging goes), it can become a problem when they wash with harsh soaps which will strip the natural oil completely. While this may feel good initially because of the immediate oil-free texture, the skin's natural response is to fire up oil production to compensate, thereby resulting in oily skin.

Balance is key. And when you are using incorrect or poor-quality products, you have no real way of knowing what the natural condition of your skin would be if you were using products that are suitable for you.

Salespeople who work behind skin care counters at your favorite department stores typically are not trained estheticians. That's not to say that once in a while you won't encounter a salesperson who does actually hold an esthetician license. But because of the rapid speed with which esthetics advances these days, simply being licensed is not enough, especially in states where there are no continuing education requirements for estheticians.

At department stores, grocery stores and drug stores, there is no proper detailed intake procedure, nor does the sales staff have the skills and tools to accurately evaluate your skin as a qualified esthetician would do. For salespeople, the only source of information about the current state of your skin is YOU, and often the condition of your skin is related to the fact that you are not currently using the right products.

Conversely, not only will a qualified esthetician be trained very well in product knowledge and skin analysis, but they will also have access to higher-quality products with stronger active ingredients, thereby resulting in much more significant results.

This brings me to prices of skin care products. It is shocking how expensive some of these non-professional skin care products can be. Published studies have shown that a $500 department store moisturizer does no better than an inexpensive drug store product. And most people don't even realize that professional skin care products provided by an esthetician are of much better-quality and are more affordable than either of those over-the-counter options.

> **Professional skin care products produce optimum results only when recommended and sold by trained skincare professionals who understand their clients' skin care needs, and have received proper training on any professional skin care line that they use and sell.**

Many of the professional skin care products used in an esthetician's treatment room and retailed by estheticians are not sold in retail stores or online. That being said, these days it is very hard for the manufacturers to control this restriction, so more and more often you will see these products being sold online...which brings us to Product Diversion.

What is Product Diversion?
Product Diversion refers to products that are being sold outside the authorized distribution channel.

The popularity of the skin care business and the evolution of the internet have created a huge problem which targets the online shopper. The methods of Product Diversion are varied. For example: A wholesale client legally orders product from a manufacturer of professional skin care products with the intent to sell them as retail products. And because many manufacturers have minimum order requirements, often the wholesale client is not able to sell their entire inventory before the products become stale or expire. At that point, the wholesaler's options are to sell the stale or expired products on eBay or Amazon or off-load the products to a third party, all of which is without the manufacturer's consent.

Other possibilities are more sinister, such as the possibility that the diverted products may have been stolen or could be the result of fraud. Diverted products can be counterfeit, diluted or altered in some way. There could be fillers added, the products could be stale or expired. There could even be a completely different product inside the bottle other than what is indicated on the label. At this writing, there really are no laws to protect consumers against Product Diversion.

Your skin is your body's largest and fastest-growing organ and it protects everything inside you, from your heart and lungs to your blood and muscles. Using a diverted product could result in irritation, infection or worse. You wouldn't risk the health of your body by purchasing discounted medications online, and you shouldn't risk the health of your skin by purchasing potentially diverted skin care products.

Over-The-Counter ("OTC")
Before I became a skin care professional, I too was an OTC shopper. I remember the day that I got my first skin care advice. I was at a department store and somehow ended up at the **** counter. *(Names have been withheld to protect the guilty.)*

I was in my early 20s and was probably using drug store products on my face at the time, because I didn't know any better. The salesperson behind the counter asked me about my skin. I told her I thought my skin was probably normal except that I had occasional breakouts.

Based upon my interpretation of my skin condition and her lack of training, she sold me several products. As I recall, I spent over $300 and I was really excited about my purchase because I had heard of the brand on television. Not only that, but everything was packaged beautifully and I got a free gift with my purchase! It was a big deal for me and I put a lot of faith in those products. As you can probably guess, not only did the products *not* improve my skin, but the breakouts increased. Looking back, the glaring errors were that exfoliation – as important as it is – was not even mentioned to me, and I had been sold a creamy cleanser and overly-rich moisturizers, which was not what I needed at that time.

After I became a trained and qualified skin care specialist, it was easy for me to look back and identify the common mistakes made by that salesperson. But I need to state clearly that it was not her fault. She was not a trained skin care professional and she didn't profess to be. She was a salesperson who was doing her job -- which was to sell products. So I am not blaming her. I am only using this example to point out that we as consumers need to qualify the information that is being given to us, especially when we are spending money to get it.

Recently, I had another experience with a salesperson that I want to share with you because it is a very common sleight-of-hand technique often used on unsuspecting shoppers:

In the city where I live, there is a lovely shopping area that is frequented by tourists because of the ritzy stores. There is one particular beauty product store that always has a well-dressed salesperson standing in the doorway trying to lure passersby in with the offer of free samples and a free eye treatment. Sometimes it's a man and other times it's a woman, but always someone with a beautiful European accent.

It is especially annoying to those of us who are not tourists because we regularly walk down that street and pass by this store on our way to someplace else. And we too are accosted every single time. So it's either "no, thank you" for what seems like the millionth time; or we must make an effort to avoid that side of the street.

One time the salesman was so persistent that I decided to listen to his sales pitch without telling him that I was an esthetician. (My hope was that in the future he'd remember that he had already talked to me and would ignore me next time I walked by.) And here is how that went:

The cute salesman with the cool accent offered me a free eye treatment that he swore would take years off my eyes, make me look refreshed, etc. He applied the eye serum under one of my eyes and I immediately felt tingling. To the general public, it might seem that some great anti-wrinkle action was happening. And I suppose that is somewhat true; but as a trained esthetician, I knew that there was an ingredient in the product which is specifically intended to irritate the skin.

What happens when the skin is irritated? It swells, of course. And swelling causes the skin to stretch, thereby smoothing the wrinkles temporarily. The wrinkles aren't really gone and will once again be visible when the swelling subsides. But to the innocent consumer, they believe this is a miracle product. So the goal of this product really is to keep your skin irritated in order to swell your wrinkles repeatedly. But the long-term effect of irritation is never a good thing.

Continuing to play along, I inquired as to what the main active ingredients were in this magic eye serum (which, by the way, cost several hundred dollars). Basically, I wanted to figure out what the irritant in this product was. His answer was that the main ingredient was Hyaluronic Acid. Well, it's common knowledge that Hyaluronic Acid is an ingredient known for its hydrating properties. In other words, it does not irritate, it hydrates.

Fortunately for me, part of this salesman's technique was to place the boxed product in front of me to entice me to purchase it. Instead I picked up the box and read the label as quickly as I could before he took it from me. I was able to look at the ingredients briefly and Hyaluronic Acid was not near the top; in fact, it was mentioned way down the list of ingredients, meaning it has very little impact in this product. I pointed that out to him and repeated my request to know what the active ingredient was that "erased" my wrinkles *(wink, wink)*. But this guy had absolutely no idea about the specifics of the product that he was trying to sell.

Multi-Level Marketing ("MLM")

These are the home-party/pyramid sales people. There are lots of different companies out there and the salespeople (aka "brand partners") are indoctrinated by their leaders to be very enthusiastic; however, they are not qualified skin care specialists and therefore do not have the training to properly analyze skin and prescribe products. Their mission is to sell products, and they are simply regurgitating the company spiel with such enthusiasm that the unsuspecting consumer can't wait to whip out his or her credit card.

Part of my intake process with a new client is to find out what skin care products she is currently using at home. There is one particular MLM company that I can always predict when I see women in their 30s-50s with breakouts. *(If I had a dollar for every time I've guessed that one right...)* The sad fact is that these clients always think there is something wrong with her skin; it does not occur to her that her skin is simply reacting to the MLM products she is using. When I switch this client to professional skin care products, her skin bounces back almost immediately.

TV and Magazines

I will repeat myself again here when I say: *Effective skin care products are never one-size-fits-all*. You cannot allow yourself to believe that a product line being hawked by a celebrity or a dermatologist is going to be right for everybody. It just doesn't work that way. These people who are trying to sell you products have not even seen you in person, so you are left to diagnose your own skin condition which will likely lead you astray.

The bottom line is that a detailed history must be taken and a proper skin analysis must be performed by a trained professional before skin care products that are best for you can be determined and recommended. And even then, things will change throughout your life and adjustments must be made to continue good skin health.

*The grass is always greener
where you water it.*

4. THE FORMULA

Home Care

There really is a formula that we all should follow to obtain optimal skin care results, even though the products and tools we each use will vary. For example, the top layers of skin, known collectively as the epidermis, is the area that estheticians are licensed to address; whereas the layers below, known as the dermis, are the dermatologists' domain. To give you a point of reference: If you cut your finger and blood is drawn, you have gone through the epidermis into the dermis.

Here are the general steps to a typical home care regimen:

Cleanse: We must cleanse our faces regularly, of course. It is especially necessary to remove makeup and sunscreen on a nightly basis. If you wear liquid or powder foundation, it is a good idea to wash your face twice: The first wash removes the makeup; the second wash cleanses the skin.

Exfoliate: This is SO important! The surface layer of the epidermis is known as the stratum corneum, or horny layer. ("Horny" in this case means scaly.) The horny layer is composed of dead skin cells, sebum[4] and environmental debris all mixed together which forms a crust on the surface of the skin. This crust causes congestion and blockage which can result in open[5] and closed[6] comedones and can prevent proper penetration of any serums applied. So basically, your products are not doing their job, and therefore are a complete waste of time and money.

Toner: Toners are considered optional by some. The reasons one might want to use a toner are many:
- If your tap water is hard or softened, there will likely be a residue left on your skin after you rinse your face. Toner on a cotton ball can remove the residue, allowing the serum that follows to penetrate effectively. A visual example of this would be to take note of the residue that is left on your shower doors. The identical residue from that same water will be left on your face after washing or rinsing, rendering your skin care products less effective.
- If you wash and condition your hair in the shower, odds are that you will have residue from your conditioner left on your face. Conditioner is made to coat hair and since you naturally have hair on your face (and back, etc.), conditioner will coat that hair as well, which may cause congestion. Toner on a cotton ball will remove that residue.
- If you struggle with acne, some toners are formulated with precise ingredients to address this issue.
- If you struggle with dry skin, some toners are formulated with ingredients to hydrate.
- Some suggest using toner on a cotton ball to remove any excess makeup after cleansing. However, it is my

---

[4] *Naturally-produced oil.*

[5] *aka "blackhead" pimples.*

[6] *aka "whitehead" pimples.*

belief that your cleanser should remove the makeup, even if it means washing twice.

Serums: Serums are to the skin like vitamins are to the body and are a vital part of beautiful skin.
- Serums *especially* are not a one-size-fits-all product. A good esthetician will recommend specific serums depending upon the current condition of your skin, the season, any hormonal activity, etc., and will make adjustments as the situation changes.
- Serums can do everything from hydrate, lighten dark spots, control oil production, and even slow down the aging process. Because serums are so active and produce such great results, they tend to be more expensive than cleansers and moisturizers, which do not penetrate into the skin.
- Serums recommended by a professional esthetician will be much more results-oriented than over-the-counter products, which by nature must be neutral and mild for use by the general population (so they don't hurt themselves!).

Moisturizer: Moisturizers are the icing on the beautiful cake. They do not penetrate but they do have an important role in hydrating and protecting the top layer of skin.
- In the daytime, moisturizers should contain sunscreen, unless you are using a separate sunscreen product.
- Nighttime moisturizers should not contain sunscreen but should contain whatever ingredients will meet your specific skin care goals. It is possible you may not even need a moisturizer, depending upon your serum.

Eye Cream: The eye area tends to be very delicate and should be treated as such. There are light-weight daytime eye creams and there are heavier creams for nighttime use. I suggest always applying eye products with your ring finger as it is the weakest digit and therefore the most gentle. Specific eye creams can address various issues:

- Wrinkles at the outer corner of the eye (aka "crow's feet.")
- Under-eye dark circles.
- Fine lines and wrinkles.
- Dehydration.

Lip Options: There are several lip products that can meet various needs:
- Lip plumpers – as we age, we lose fullness in our lips. There are many new professional skin care products available from your esthetician to enhance your lips without painful medical injections that can sometimes produce obvious malformations.
- Lip exfoliators – lips should be exfoliated just like the rest of your face.
- Lip treatments – to hydrate and rejuvenate.
- Sun protection – you must protect your lips. They get the same sun exposure that the rest of your face does, and therefore need the same protection. There are great lipsticks and lip glosses that contain spf, so sun protection is easy, colorful and gorgeous.

Neck and décolleté: Treat the area between your chin and your breasts the same as you would your face because it gets almost as much exposure to the sun and the environment. Sadly, the décolleté is overlooked or abused by the sun and often is the first obvious sign of aging.

Hands and arms: Also often forgotten, your hands probably get more sun exposure than any other part of your body. Unless you wear gloves or were advised long ago to put sunscreen on your hands daily, noticeable brown spots can begin to appear on your hands by age 30. And even if you do apply sunscreen to your hands, it will likely be removed with hand-washing throughout the day.

Spots on the hands are sometimes referred to as sun spots, liver spots or age spots, but most of the time it is the same hyperpigmentation typically caused by sun exposure. At some point, you may begin to see white spots replace the dark spots, which is an indication that your pigment has been depleted. Those white spots are there forever because while pigmented skin can be lightened at least somewhat, there is no esthetic treatment that can replace lack of pigment.

The Esthetician

As mentioned in an earlier chapter, consumers are bombarded with ads by skin care product retailers, as well as advertisements about medical services provided by doctors and surgeons. Those ads are on TV, in magazines, on the sides of buses and benches. On the other hand, what you won't see are big ad campaigns by estheticians, who for years have been quietly helping clients obtain their skin care goals. This imbalance puts estheticians at a disadvantage in the big business that esthetics has become.

Because rules and laws vary state-to-state, it can be hard to identify the well-trained and qualified estheticians without doing some research. (Fortunately, the internet makes that easy.) Simply holding an esthetician license is no guarantee that the person is well-trained in today's esthetics.

Another consideration is that in many states, those holding a cosmetology license are legally permitted to perform esthetic treatments even though their training programs include only a couple of days' education specifically related to esthetics. But there are exceptions. In fact, I personally know many with Cosmetologist licenses who chose to further their esthetic education and training and ultimately became excellent estheticians.

My best advice is to look for estheticians who actively continue their esthetic education by attending trade shows and post-graduate classes, as well as subscribing to trade magazines (and reading them regularly.)

Don't be afraid to try out a new esthetician because sometimes their education is more up-to-date than someone who has been a licensed esthetician for many years. Esthetics is evolving constantly, and I know from my own 17 years' experience that if I wasn't actively keeping up with technology, science and customer service, I would have been left behind long ago.

When assessing an esthetician's credentials, be mindful of the fact that in most states, the licensed titles on our licenses are "Esthetician," or in a few states it is spelled "Aesthetician." And as of this writing, there are currently only 4 states that offer a licensed title of "Master Esthetician" (or "Master Esthetician Manager"). Those four states are: DC, WA, VA and UT.

Nowhere in the United States is there currently a licensed title of "Clinical Esthetician" or "Medical Esthetician" -- even if the esthetician is working in a medical facility which is owned or managed by a medical doctor. [7] (*Use of any title other than what is on the license may be punishable by law in some states.*)

Do not assume an esthetician is more qualified or better just because she works in a doctor's medi-spa. It's just not true. I can't tell you the number of dermatologists, plastic surgeons, internists, gynecologists, dentists, etc., wanting to get into the spa/esthetics business who have contacted me over the years looking for an esthetician to hire, no experience necessary; just anybody with an esthetician license.

My opinion is that your very best source of effective skin care is a highly-educated and skilled esthetician – whether you find them in a spa, a doctor's office or a solo skin care studio.

---

[7] *National Coalition of Estheticians, Manufacturers/Distributors & Associations.*

Another obstacle to finding a good esthetician may be related to the antiquated licensing requirements in some U.S. states. However, even if some esthetician training programs are not keeping up with the rapidly-changing field of esthetics, the really good estheticians continue their education on their own and work very hard throughout their careers to keep themselves up-to-date with esthetic developments and trends.

I always suggest to estheticians that they continually update their websites with any and all continuing education they have gained and that they display their post-graduate training certificates prominently in their place of business. All of this helps consumers initially assess an esthetician's credentials and will ultimately contribute to the client's overall comfort and trust level.

Facials are workouts for the skin.

5. THE FACIAL

What is a Facial?

For some of us, we are on vacation and the spa menu is delicious and tempting and we can't resist a relaxing facial with wonderful scents in a tantalizing environment. For others, it's the day we wake up and look in the mirror and see fine lines, wrinkles and brown spots staring back at us.

You don't need me to tell you how wonderful the relaxing spa or resort facial is, so I am going to focus on the clinical aspect of skin care.

First of all, of course, "anti-aging" is a misnomer. We are going to age, there's no "anti" about it. But we do have some say about how well we do it. It is possible to slow down the process and in some cases even reverse certain aspects of visible aging. There is much that you can do, and it doesn't involve a facelift or doctor or crazy expensive products and treatments. Esthetics has advanced so much since I became an esthetician in 1999, that simple *proper* skin care can delay or even completely eliminate the desire for surgical remedies. (I just wish every woman who is concerned about signs of aging knew this!)

Facial Virgins

If you have never had a really good facial, you might imagine it to be an intimidating experience. So let me begin by giving you a glimpse into what a first-time facial might be like with a qualified and skilled professional esthetician.

Your first visit will involve an intake process in which pertinent information such as medical history, allergies, historical and current product usage, etc., will be collected from you in order to determine any possible contraindications and to ascertain the current condition of your skin. At this time, you and your esthetician can discuss any specific skin care goals you may have.

For most facials, the esthetician needs only your head and shoulders (and sometimes your arms) uncovered. You will be asked to change into a facial gown or wrap and will be offered instructions regarding how the facial wrap is to be worn, where to hang your clothes and place your jewelry and shoes. Often, clients will remove everything except their underwear, but of course your personal level of comfort dictates which items of clothing you will leave underneath the facial wrap.

Which brings me to a story that will reveal why I always recommend to estheticians that they go into great detail with first-time clients regarding the disrobing process:

When I owned my spa many years ago, we offered back waxing for men. For this service, the only disrobing that is required is the removal of the shirt; however, we had men's wraps available which attached at the waist, leaving the upper torso exposed.

I had one particular new client who had been referred to me for back waxing. As always, after explaining the procedure to the new male client, I left the room to give him privacy so he could get comfortable lying face-down on my treatment table.

As is my habit, I knocked on the door to the treatment room before entering and inquired if he was ready for me to enter the room. He replied that yes, he was. So I opened the door. And there he was completely naked -- not lying face-down on the treatment table, but standing next to it. As I recall, he explained that he was attempting to adjust the treatment table, for some reason (which was not necessary since I had already positioned the table properly).
Being the Zen-Goddess that I pretend to be at all times, I calmly requested that he lie face-down on the treatment table. I covered his lower body with a towel, and I proceeded with the wax service.

This client came in again a month or so later, and this time one of my other estheticians was assigned to him. She was aware of the situation so she made it abundantly clear what our disrobing protocol was. And he completely ignored it again. The odd thing was that he was a really nice young man; he had just moved to the area and he swore that he had been having his back waxed for years. But apparently his former esthetician's disrobing preferences were different than ours. So because he made my employees uncomfortable by not adhering to our rules, I had to fire him as a client.

Okay, back to facials...

At each appointment, your skin will be completely cleansed and a detailed evaluation will be performed, utilizing various esthetic tools including a lighted magnifying lamp. Typically, the consultation will be more lengthy and detailed during your first appointment, as it is a very important step that allows the esthetician to determine how best to meet your skin's needs and to help you reach whatever your goals may be.

Especially during the first appointment, your esthetician will communicate with you throughout the facial to whatever degree is appropriate for the type of facial service you are having. This is so that you will understand the current condition of your skin and the products, procedures and tools that are being used during the treatment, as well as to ascertain your comfort level at all times. You, of course, are free to ask any questions and discuss anything with your esthetician at any time during the facial.

A good esthetician will make recommendations as to proper home care to extend the life of the facial and to achieve optimum skin health. But it's important to remember that the esthetician can only do 50% of the work in the treatment room to achieve a client's skin care goals. The other half depends upon the client's willingness to do her part at home. In other words, an esthetician cannot do more for the client than the client is willing to do for herself.

> **Not one esthetician that I know of got into this business to work as a salesperson with the primary goal being to sell skin care products. However, it is an important part of an esthetician's job to offer clients appropriate home care products which will extend the benefits of the facial and help them to achieve and maintain optimum skin health.**

Skin care products are ever-evolving and just keep getting better and better, and a good esthetician keeps up with of all of that so you don't have to. Your esthetician's expertise is vital to your good skin health and is essential to the return and retention of your youthful glow.

Estheticians are trained to use esthetic tools and active products in their treatment rooms which are not approved for client's home use. So without question, the best thing you can do for your skin is to find a qualified esthetician and have regular facials once a month, every six weeks, quarterly (or whatever works best for you), provided you are also using professional products at home as recommended by your esthetician. If you are having any particular skin issues, your esthetician may recommend coming in more frequently until the problem is under control, and then you can cut back to a maintenance schedule.

There are, of course, many reasons why women might not wish to have regular facials. It might be a financial issue or a time constraint issue. Or it could simply be a matter of personal comfort.[8] In any case, these are all very understandable scenarios. But at the very least, you should have an initial consultation with a qualified esthetician so that he or she can properly evaluate your skin and ascertain the important information necessary to recommend a specific home care protocol for you.

It is also wise to have follow-up consultations with your esthetician as often as possible so that he or she can adjust your home care protocol based upon changes in your skin related to hormonal fluctuations, stress level, environment, and life in general.

The Tools
Some of the tools a properly trained and qualified esthetician might use to assess your current skin condition are:

- Magnifying Lamp
- Moisture Checker
- Skin Scope
- Woods Lamp
- pH Pencil
- Glogau Scale – *Classification of Photo Age Groups based upon a client's aging analysis and photo damage associated with UV radiation exposure as indicators for skin condition.*

---

[8] *Some women are uncomfortable without their makeup. However, there is often an opportunity to reapply your makeup before you leave the facial room. Also, many estheticians retail mineral makeup and sometimes will apply it for you after the facial.*

- Fitzpatrick Scale – *Based upon basal skin color and the skin's response to ultraviolet radiation exposure. The Fitzpatrick Skin type/Classification presents a useful scale to determine sensitivity levels based on pigmentation and sensitivity to UV radiation exposure.*

Just as the services offered by estheticians will vary from facials designed to pamper, all the way to highly-clinical esthetic treatments, there are also many different tools that we may use. But because the laws governing estheticians vary state-to-state, it is not possible for me to list every piece of esthetic equipment that a licensed esthetician is legally allowed to use in the treatment room. So the sampling below is not intended to be comprehensive; rather, it is designed to give those of you who may be "Facial Virgins" a general idea of the esthetic tools a properly trained and qualified esthetician might use to maximize your skin care:

- Microdermabrasion
- Ultrasonic
- Ultrasound
- Skin Spatula
- High Frequency Current
- Galvanic Current
- Microcurrent
- LED (Light Emitting Diodes)
- Rotary Brush
- Steamer
- Vacuum/Spray

*Improve your selfies.
See an esthetician.*

The 7 Witches of Menopause:

Itchy, Bitchy, Sweaty, Sleepy, Bloated, Forgetful and Psycho.

6. SKIN CONDITIONS

Teen Acne

Although a good diet is important to overall health, acne is not caused by eating chocolate or French fries, contrary to popular belief. Acne typically runs in families, and teen acne is often a result of fluctuating hormones related to puberty. Although teen acne is sometimes hard to control completely until the hormones settle down, proper home care in conjunction with acne services performed by a qualified esthetician can make a huge difference; and quite possibly can eliminate the need for prescription medication. If the esthetician determines that the teen acne is of a more severe grade, he or she can refer to a dermatologist that specializes in acne.

It is wise to address teen acne very quickly, as ignoring it will likely increase the severity and can result in scarring, not to mention the emotional and psychological toll that often accompanies teenage acne. Many boys' acne will continue until about age 23, 24 or longer. Girls' acne may continue considerably longer.[9]

---

[9] James E. Fulton Jr., M.D., Ph.D., *Acne Rx*

Recent research supports the theory that hormones injected into dairy cows can exacerbate teen acne. The use of genetically-engineered Recombinant Bovine Growth Hormone (rBGH/rBST) in dairy cows was approved by the Food & Drug Administration in late 1993 and has been used since 1994.

When rBGH gets injected into dairy cows, milk production is increased and some believe this is the explanation for earlier menstruation in girls and increased height in boys. Ingestion of growth hormones in dairy can be avoided by consuming organic dairy products. The good news is that although rBGH is still legal in the U.S., many major grocery stores no longer sell milk from injected cows.

Accutane. I urge you to do extensive research before opting for aggressive prescription medication such as Accutane and its derivatives to control acne. While it is often successful at controlling acne, the side effects and long-term effects can be serious.

Hormonal Acne

Women are often surprised and puzzled when they suddenly get a bout of acne when they are in their 30s and 40s. The inflammation often appears in the jaw and chin area and can be very painful. This is related to pre-menopausal hormone activity, and proper exfoliation is vital. It is essential to visit your esthetician ASAP for treatments and an adjustment to your prescribed daily home care products to keep the breakouts under control.

Other Causes of Acne

There are a multitude of reasons we might break out occasionally such as a reaction to certain cosmetics, or neglecting to wash makeup or sunscreen off of our face at night. I have seen areas of congestion caused by clients repeatedly resting their chin in their hands or from frequent wearing of a visor or cap. I've even had a client whose lower face was breaking out due to regular licks of love from her dog. Estheticians are trained to determine the cause and recommend treatments and/or products to resolve the specific problem.

Rosacea

Rosacea is a common but poorly understood disorder of the facial skin that is estimated to affect well over 16 million Americans -- and most of them don't know it. In fact, while Rosacea is becoming increasingly widespread as the populous Baby Boom generation enters the most susceptible ages, a Gallup survey found that 95 percent of Americans had known little or nothing about the signs or symptoms prior to their Rosacea diagnosis.

Rosacea cannot be cured, but it can be controlled. Because of its red-faced, acne-like effects on personal appearance, it can cause significant psychological, social and occupational problems if left untreated. [10]

Men's Skin Care

When it comes to skin care, men are great clients. All they ask for is an understanding of the principles of proper skin care, simple treatments, and clear instructions regarding use of their products. Their simple requests are to provide them with written literature and keep the number of products to a minimum, please. Give them that, and they will be compliant and loyal clients.

The one problematic issue for men is their reluctance to regularly use sunscreen. A fact from the American Cancer Society: *From ages 15-39, men are 55 percent more likely to die of melanoma than women in the same age group.*

Men's skin typically tends to be thicker and oilier than the average woman's skin due to the predominance of male hormones. Oftentimes men do not realize that they are

---

[10] *www.rosacea.org*

41

exacerbating their oily skin issue by constantly trying to wash away the excess oil with hand or body soap, which actually makes the condition worse. I know a man who occasionally felt so oily that he would wash his face with just about anything, including soap from the dispenser in a public restroom. Once I got him on the proper maintenance products, his skin immediately normalized.

Some men have bouts of skin irritation, known as folliculitis, in the areas where they shave. A qualified esthetician can remedy this problem by way of specific treatments and home care product recommendations.

*Wrinkles merely indicate
where smiles have been.*

~ Mark Twain

Go braless...

it pulls the wrinkles from your face.

7. ZERO TO FACELIFT

It's tragic to me – and I see it all the time – how often women go from no proper skin care at all directly to a facelift, without even knowing about the many state-of-the-art youthful aging solutions that are available through a qualified esthetician. There is a vast array of products and treatments that should be explored before risking one's safety by turning to overly-aggressive procedures and elective surgery.

Because there are so many levels of skin care and esthetic treatments available, it can be difficult for the average consumer to sift through so much incorrect and misleading information found online. Estheticians were around long before doctors jumped into the "spa" business with their creation of the Medical Spa. To assume that a medical facility is a better choice for skin care is not necessarily accurate. This is evidenced by doctors who readily recommend or hand out samples of low-quality over-the-counter soaps and other products, or the other extreme of defaulting to aggressive medications and treatments that may not be necessary.

Keep in mind that if you go to a medical doctor's "medi-spa" for skin care, often their goal is to lead you down the road to medical products and procedures. Similarly, if you look to a plastic surgeon for skin care, that road will likely lead to surgical procedures. I am certainly not saying that these options are bad ones, because I believe there is room for all of us in the world of skin care. However, there are a lot of gentler options that I think are a better place to start your journey to youthful aging.

Facelift Financials
Here are some financial statistics for you to consider about the facelift, according to 2014 statistics from the American Society of Plastic Surgeons:

*The **average cost of a facelift is $6,550.** When you are calculating the cost of your facelift surgery, keep in mind that these prices are only for the plastic surgeon's fee and do not include the costs for the surgical facility, the anesthesia, the surgical chin strap, prescription medicine, or any tests that may be needed. And it's important to take into consideration that most health insurance does not cover facelift surgery or its complications.*

*Wrinkles mean you **laughed**,*
*Gray hairs means you **cared**,*
*And scars mean you **lived**!*

Pale? I'm not pale.

It's called porcelain,
and I'm rocking it!

8. THE SUN

The Magic Potion

The Fountain of Youth does exist and it is called *sunscreen*. Sunscreen is the cheapest and best anti-aging tool on the market today. But there is one catch: *You must use it!*

To emphasize this point, here is a visual for you: Raise your arm up and take a look at your underarm skin just below your armpit. Now compare the color and texture you see there to the topside of your forearm which is regularly exposed to the sun. Notice any difference?

Let's take it one step further. Take a peek at your derriere. Unless you have spent a lot of time over the years sunning yourself at a nude beach, the skin in that area should be just about pristine in color. And for even further proof, if you have access to the fanny of an elderly person, take a look there too. It's probably spot-free. Age doesn't matter; it's all about sun exposure.

> **Some will argue that sunscreen prevents us from obtaining our much-needed vitamin D; however, researchers will argue that you can get a sufficient dose of Vitamin D right through the hair on your head.**

Can you imagine in what perfect condition your face would be if you had consistently been applying sunscreen since you were a child? You would look a decade or two younger than your counterparts who were not regular sunscreen-wearers.

Sunscreens have evolved from the gooey white stuff of yesteryear that you bought over-the-counter at the drug store or grocery store, to glorious facial products with fabulous ingredients that do wonderful things for your skin. From your esthetician, you can purchase a virtual wardrobe of sunscreens. There are tinted sunscreens that come in many shades; there are oil-free sunscreens, organic sunscreens, and hydrating sunscreens; there are water-resistant sunscreens for water sports and other athletic activities, and there are luxurious sunscreens for everyday use that include moisturizers, peptides[11] and antioxidants.[12]

The good news is that people have become more aware of the dangers of the sun in recent years, so they have gotten better at applying sunscreen when they will be participating in full sun activities. However, they still do not completely grasp how important daily sunscreen really is.

---

[11] *Science has proven that peptides can reduce wrinkles in your skin and reverse the signs of aging.*

[12] *Antioxidants are nutrients (vitamins and minerals) and enzymes (proteins inside your body) that can help to prevent and repair damage to your body's tissue. If you've seen a peeled apple turn brown, you've seen oxidation in action.*

Frequently, people who drive a lot will have more sun damage on the left side (driver's side) of their face than on the right side. And unless you are wearing driving gloves or sunscreen on your hands, you will eventually begin to see brown spots (hyperpigmentation) where the sun targets your hands through your windshield.

Change Your Evil Rays

The difference between the two most commonly-known Ultraviolet Rays is that UVA is what causes aging and UVB is what causes sunburn. It's easy to remember it this way:

UV**A** = **A**ging
UV**B** = **B**urning

A qualified esthetician will assist you with the sunscreens you'll need based upon your skin type and your lifestyle, and will give you instructions for proper use and storage.

Warning signs: The ABCDEs of Melanoma

Moles, brown spots and growths on the skin are usually harmless — but not always. Anyone who has more than 100 moles is at greater risk for melanoma. The first signs can appear in one or more atypical moles. That's why it's so important to get to know your skin very well and to recognize any changes in the moles on your body. Look for the ABCDE signs of melanoma, and if you see one or more, make an appointment with a physician immediately.

A. **ASYMMETRY** - If you draw a line through the middle of a benign mole, the two sides will match, meaning it is symmetrical. If, however, you draw a line through this mole, the two halves will not match, meaning it is asymmetrical; a warning sign for melanoma.
B. **BORDERS** - A benign mole has smooth, even borders, unlike melanomas. The borders of an early melanoma

tend to be uneven. The edges may be scalloped or notched.

C. **COLOR** - Most benign moles are all one color — often a single shade of brown. Having a variety of colors is another warning signal. A number of different shades of brown, tan or black could appear. A melanoma may also become red, white or blue.

D. **DIAMETER** - Benign moles usually have a **smaller diameter** than malignant ones. Melanomas usually are larger in **diameter** than the eraser on your pencil tip (¼ inch or 6mm), but they may sometimes be smaller when first detected.

E. **EVOLVING** - Common, benign moles look the same over time. Be on the alert when a mole starts to **evolve or change** in any way. When a mole is **evolving**, see a doctor. Any change — in size, shape, color, elevation, or another trait, or any new symptom such as bleeding, itching or crusting — points to danger.

Here are some statistics from the Skin Cancer Foundation website:

GENERAL
- Each year there are more new cases of skin cancer than the combined incidence of cancers of the breast, prostate, lung and colon.
- Each year in the U.S. over 5.4 million cases of non-melanoma skin cancer are treated in more than 3.3 million people.
- Over the past 3 decades, more people have had skin cancer than all other cancers combined.
- One in five Americans will develop skin cancer in the course of a lifetime.
- Between 40 and 50 percent of Americans who live to age 65 will have either basal cell carcinoma or squamous cell carcinoma at least once.

- Basal cell carcinoma (BCC) is the most common form of skin cancer. BCCs are rarely fatal, but can be highly disfiguring if allowed to grow.
- Squamous cell carcinoma (SCC) is the second most common form of skin cancer.
- Organ transplant patients are approximately 100 times more likely than the general public to develop squamous cell carcinoma.
- Actinic Keratosis is the most common precancer; it affects more than 58 million Americans.
- About 90 percent of non-melanoma skin cancers are associated with exposure to ultraviolet (UV) radiation from the sun.
- The annual cost of treating skin cancers in the U.S. is estimated at $8.1 billion: about $4.8 billion for non-melanoma skin cancers and $3.3 billion for melanoma.

MELANOMA

- One person dies of melanoma every hour (every 52 minutes).
- An estimated 76,380 new cases of invasive melanoma will be diagnosed in the U.S. in 2016.
- Melanoma accounts for less than one percent of skin cancer cases, but the vast majority of skin cancer deaths.
- On average, a person's risk for melanoma doubles if he or she has had more than five sunburns.
- Regular daily use of an SPF 15 or higher sunscreen reduces the risk of developing squamous cell carcinoma by about 40 percent[16] and the risk of developing melanoma by 50 percent.
- Melanoma is the most common form of cancer for young adults 25-29 years old and the second most common form of cancer for young people 15-29 years old.
- The estimated 5-year survival rate for patients whose melanoma is detected early is about 98 percent in the U.S. The survival rate falls to 63 percent when the

disease reaches the lymph nodes, and 17 percent when the disease metastasizes to distant organs.

- Melanoma is one of only three cancers with an increasing mortality rate for men, along with liver cancer and esophageal cancer.
- An estimated 10,130 people will die of melanoma in 2016.
- The vast majority of melanomas are caused by the sun. In fact, one UK study found that about 86 percent of melanomas can be attributed to exposure to ultraviolet (UV) radiation from the sun.

MEN/WOMEN
- An estimated 46,870 new cases of invasive melanoma in men and 29,510 in women will be diagnosed in the U.S. in 2016.
- An estimated 6,750 men and 3,380 women in the U.S. will die from melanoma in 2016.
- From ages 15-39, men are 55 percent more likely to die of melanoma than women in the same age group.
- Up until age 49, significantly more women develop melanoma than men (1 in 206 women vs. 1 in 297 men). From age 50 on, significantly more men develop melanoma than women. Overall, one in 33 men and one in 52 women will develop melanoma in their lifetimes.
- Women aged 49 and under have a higher probability of developing melanoma than any other cancer except breast and thyroid cancers.

INDOOR TANNING
- Ultraviolet radiation (UVR) is a proven human carcinogen.
- As of September 2, 2014, ultraviolet (UV) tanning devices were reclassified by the FDA from Class I (low risk), to Class II (moderate risk) devices.
- The International Agency for Research on Cancer, an affiliate of the World Health Organization, includes ultraviolet (UV) tanning devices in its Group 1, a list of agents that are cancer-causing to humans. Group 1 also

includes agents such as plutonium, cigarettes, and solar UV radiation.

- Eleven states plus the District of Columbia now prohibit indoor tanning for minors younger than age 18: California, Delaware, Hawaii, Illinois, Louisiana, Minnesota, Nevada, New Hampshire, North Carolina, Texas and Vermont. Oregon and Washington prohibit minors under age 18 from using indoor tanning devices, unless a prescription is provided.
- Brazil and Australia have banned indoor tanning altogether. Austria, Belgium, Finland, France, Germany, Iceland, Italy, Norway, Portugal, Spain and the United Kingdom have banned indoor tanning for people younger than age 18.
- More than 419,000 cases of skin cancer in the U.S. each year are linked to indoor tanning, including about 245,000 basal cell carcinomas, 168,000 squamous cell carcinomas, and 6,200 melanomas.
- More people develop skin cancer because of tanning than develop lung cancer because of smoking.
- Those who have ever tanned indoors have a 67 percent increased risk of developing squamous cell carcinoma and a 29 percent increased risk of developing basal cell carcinoma.
- Those who have ever tanned indoors have a 69 percent risk of developing basal cell carcinoma before age 40.
- Individuals who have used tanning beds 10 or more times in their lives have a 34 percent increased risk of developing melanoma compared to those who have never used tanning beds.
- People who first use a tanning bed before age 35 increase their risk for melanoma by 75 percent.

PEDIATRICS

- Melanoma accounts for up to three percent of all pediatric cancers.
- The treatment of childhood melanoma is often delayed due to misdiagnosis of pigmented lesions, which occurs up to 40 percent of the time.

ETHNICITY

- Skin cancer comprises one to two percent of all cancers in blacks and Asian Indians.
- The estimated 5-year melanoma survival rate for blacks is only 70 percent, versus 93 percent for whites.
- Late-stage melanoma diagnoses are more prevalent among minority patients than Caucasian patients; 52 percent of non-Hispanic black patients and 26 percent of Hispanic patients receive an initial diagnosis of advanced stage melanoma, versus 16 percent of non-Hispanic white patients.
- Melanomas in blacks, Asians, Filipinos, Indonesians, and native Hawaiians most often occur on non-exposed skin with less pigment, with up to 60-75 percent of tumors arising on the palms, soles, mucous membranes and nail regions.
- Basal cell carcinoma is the most common cancer in Caucasians, Hispanics, Chinese Asians and the Japanese.
- Squamous cell carcinoma (SCC) is the most common skin cancer among blacks and Asian Indians.
- Squamous cell carcinomas in blacks tend to be more aggressive and are associated with a 20-40 percent risk of metastasis (spreading).
- Skin cancer represents approximately 2-4 percent of all cancers in Asians.

SKIN AGING

- An estimated 90 percent of skin aging is caused by the sun.
- People who use sunscreen with an SPF of 15 or higher daily show 24 percent less skin aging than those who do not use sunscreen daily.
- Sun damage is cumulative. Only about 23 percent of lifetime exposure occurs by age 18.

*I finally figured out
my eyebrows.*

They're sisters, not twins.

9. HAIR REMOVAL

Women have a soft hair over most of their bodies, including their faces. This hair is known as vellus hair. It is a non-issue to some and bothersome to others. There are many ways to remove unwanted facial hair, be it the soft vellus hair or shaping of the brows. Please don't be persuaded by the Old Wives' Tale that removing facial hair will cause it to grow back thicker and darker. It is not true. In fact, I can tell you from personal experience that the opposite is true. For example, those women who followed the skinny eyebrow trend years ago have major regrets about that choice because that hair did not grow back at all. Regretfully, they are stuck with those skinny brows forever while the trend has moved on to a more natural brow.

Waxing
There are many methods of hair removal and varying opinions about them all. I waxed body parts for many years and here is what I can tell you from my own personal experience:

What you must know before you go
Licensed waxers are a must! The most important statement I can make on this issue is to get your waxing done by a licensed professional. In California, for example, there is a

huge problem with waxing being performed illegally in nail salons. Only licensed Cosmetologists and Estheticians are legally permitted to perform waxing services in California. Manicurists are not. This is a safety issue, so please be certain that whomever is doing your waxing is legally allowed to perform those services in your state. *(Check your state's licensing board's website.)*

Using the state of California as an example once again, the law is that the technician's license *"shall be conspicuously posted at their primary work station."*[13] Check the laws in your state, and if you don't see the technician's license, ask for it. If they don't have the proper license, then it's doubtful that they are properly trained, especially in sanitation and disinfection practices which can be a major health and safety issue.

Double-dipping is dangerous! For those who are not familiar with this term, let me explain: The waxer should use *one* disposable stick per dip into the wax pot. In other words, dip it once, apply the wax to the client, *throw the stick away*. And repeat, repeat, repeat -- as many times, and with as many sticks, as it takes to complete the wax service.

To emphasize just how important the "no double-dipping" rule is, here is a visual for you:

Imagine that the double-dipping waxer who is about to wax your lip dips her waxing stick into her wax pot. As she pulls the stick back out of the wax pot, there is a residual pubic hair from her previous client's bikini wax attached. Do you want that wax stick anywhere near your lip? I think not! And besides pubic hair and skin cells, think of the bacteria that could be in the wax pot from previous clients' feces, urine, and whatever else.

---

[13] CA Board of Cosmetology, (Article 9, *Licenses,* Section 965)

In order to determine whether a waxer double-dips or not, don't bother to call ahead and ask. That could simply result in him or her not double-dipping in front of you, but that doesn't change what is already marinating in that wax pot from clients who came before you. Instead, look for signs such as a dirty wax pot, the waxer using non-disposable wax sticks, or perhaps not seeing or hearing them throw away a wax stick after each dip into the pot.

Types of Wax

There are two types of wax that estheticians typically use in the treatment room. One is often referred to as soft wax, which is typically removed with a cloth or pellon strip. Soft wax is often used for waxing larger body parts such as legs. The other type of wax is commonly known as hard wax and is often used for facial waxing. Many estheticians use a combination of both waxes for various hair removal services.

Pre- and Post-wax

For optimal results, at least 3 weeks outgrowth of hair is suggested in most cases, depending upon the area to be waxed. Sometimes an esthetician might want to prepare the skin before waxing, in which case a cleanser or prep oil will be used. For bikini waxes or men's chest or back waxing, trimming of extremely long hairs is sometimes necessary as it will result in a more comfortable waxing experience; but it may slow down the service. So, of course, maintaining a regular hair removal schedule is preferred as it will make the process quicker and easier for both the client and the esthetician.

It is often requested (and always appreciated) that clients freshen up their private areas before coming in for any body hair removal services.

Post-wax, estheticians will usually apply some sort of calming product or possibly an antiseptic product or high-frequency treatment to prevent bumps that often appear with a first-time wax, especially in the lip or bikini area.

Ouch!?

It has been my experience that most people happily discover that waxing done by a really well-trained esthetician is much less painful than they had feared. There are also products that clients can purchase for home use and apply to the area shortly before the waxing appointment. This process will numb the area, thereby resulting in a more comfortable waxing experience.

Sugaring

Gaining in popularity is hair removal by a technique known as sugaring. Sugaring paste is hypoallergenic[14] and non-comedogenic[15] and will not adhere to live skin cells, which means it causes less trauma to the skin than other forms of hair removal. Sugar paste is never hot and therefore will not burn the skin. And there is no sharing of the sugar paste among clients, so no double-dipping is involved. The sugar paste will rinse clean with warm water, and no residue will be left on the skin.

I refuse to see them as chin hairs.
We shall call them stray eyebrows.

---

[14] *Unlikely to cause an allergic reaction.*

[15] *Unlikely to cause skin breakouts.*

AFTERWORD

I am certainly not suggesting that aggressive medical esthetic treatments and surgical remedies are a bad thing. I am only suggesting that you take the care of your skin and the process of your aging into your own hands. This means you educate yourself on ALL of your options before committing to something expensive, irreversible and possibly dangerous. There is an enormous and constantly evolving menu of options that a well-trained esthetician can offer you; and in my opinion, that is the best (and safest) place to start your skin care journey.

For those of you who have hesitated to have a facial, or have had a flawed facial experience, I urge you to give it another try. Esthetics has advanced from the "steam & cream" beauty treatments of yesterday to the clinical, results-oriented facial services of today. It doesn't matter if you are in your twenties or on the other side of menopause, please use the tips I have given in this book to find a qualified esthetician in your area and give him or her a try.

Great estheticians are educated and trained to provide you with the exact services and products that can transform your skin, no matter what your starting point may be. That is the real reason estheticians are in this business; it brings us great joy to help you look good and feel better.

ABOUT THE AUTHOR

Diane Buccola is the owner of SpaBizBoard.com, a popular message board and learning tool for the spa industry which she created in 2006, long before Facebook and other of today's social media sites became popular. Estheticians and spa professionals from all over the world have contributed to SpaBizBoard over the last decade which has created a vast database of knowledge, none of which is accessible to the general public.

In her continuing effort to raise the standards of esthetics, Diane serves on the Les Nouvelles Esthetiques & Spa Magazine Advisory Board and is a well-respected author and speaker at International Congress of Esthetics & Spa events throughout the U.S. Diane has written two books; one for the spa trade, *The Heart of Esthetics: Creating Loyal Clientele and Achieving Financial Success,* and *Estheticians Are a Girl's Best Friend,* which is for consumers and is designed to help them navigate the world of esthetics and skin care.

Diane obtained her esthetician license in the state of California in 1999 and shortly thereafter opened a day spa. After selling her day spa several years later, she opened a solo practice which allows her more time to work as a consultant, trainer and mentor for estheticians. One year after the NCEA Certified Professional Esthetician[16] certification became available, Diane met the qualifications to become NCEA Certified in 2008. Not only are the successful candidates required to pass a grueling written exam, but they must also maintain certification in First Aid, CPR and AED[17] and must meet continuing education requirements in order to renew their NCEA Certification.

---

[16] *www.NCEAcertified.tv*

[17] *Automated External Defibrillator*

Be your own kind of beautiful.